SECRETS TO HEALTH WELLNESS

TABLE OF CONTENTS

INTRODUCTION

While starting a wellness program may appear to be a challenging job, and it is not. It is just like a carefully orchestrated mechanism to allow individuals to improve power and enhance their wellbeing. For this, good health education and suitable medical screenings need to be provided to individuals. Such initiatives often observed in large corporations and businesses need the first groundwork environment for the employee and executive consultation and approval. An efficient and successful program can be achieved. To ensure health-related alertness among individuals, several activities such as health counseling, health fairs, on-site fitness services, weight loss programs, medical screenings, nutrition education, stress management, and free health care programs, including some tests such as pH, blood pressure, and blood sugar level tests, are typically carried out.

Tests are used in some health wellness services to identify illnesses early. The motto is that prevention is superior to cure. vaccines, child health care, ill effects of alcohol and smoking, and maternal health are all made known to individuals. Typically, individuals neglect minor health-related conditions, making room for larger ailments. Only through proper health education can such problems be removed. In the long run, minor symptoms can lead to serious health problems. Precautionary steps must therefore be taken to create awareness among individuals to motivate them to remain fit.

Employees in a company are typically the subject of health programs that focus on stress management. Big organizations and medium-scale enterprises are also involved in raising consciousness among their staff about health. The results positively affect the bottom line and provide workers with a range of stress-reduction options, called Stress Buster. Stress is the most important factor to consider since it can be found in almost every part of an organization; thus, qualitative steps to minimize it are required. Group events also create a positive atmosphere and enhance employee relations, promoting mutual respect and understanding, among other things. Because of their successful and genuine outcomes, corporate health care services are

a success with businesses. Employees' confidence is reduced, and their productivity is improved as a result of such health services.

A sound working environment is often easier, whether it is an entity or a community. It can step together for a mutual purpose when a nation is fit.

CHAPTER 1:

OUR HEALTH WELL

"We cannot grow unless we change. We are not living if we do not grow. Development necessitates a temporary loss of security." This could not have been saying better by Gail Sheehy. We thrive on protection as women. In our relationships, in our friendships, our finances, and our hearts, we crave it. An inherent drive resides inside the comfort to say "It's all fine" at the end of the day. We want to have all of this and do all of it, but sometimes, the ambition comes with a price that we pay and don't even know it.

You see, the beauty and intention of saying that we have it all are to enjoy it once we get there as well. Yeah, we know that we will never truly arrive because our lives are a journey and not a destination, but don't we all want to be able to say that we are

enjoying that journey at some point? The reality is that we seldom confess to having this feeling. If we do, it's usually over dinner with the girls or in themiddle of our silent, screaming thoughts. We want it, but we don't think we can.

We must learn to cultivate our wellbeing as women! In the adverbial sense and the noun sense, I use it well; the adverb means that we need to learn the art of creating a sustainable space in our full, busy schedules to ensure that we remain dedicated and strong on the journey. No one leaves unprepared

on a trip who genuinely loves the destination—as women, knowing what we need to offer on an ongoing basis is critical for our colleagues, our spouses, friends, and society. For others, an hour-long massage every two weeks can suffice. It could be a trip to the lake with others or a full weekend of shopping alone. Learn to cultivate, defend, and most importantly, claim whatever it is that you crave. We have the right to preserve our health as earth's mothers, as women among men, as husbands, sisters, daughters, and lovers.

Woman, we are reservoirs, you and I. We are the wells that continually give, offer, and sustain life to all who come to us. But what good is a well if it runs dry for anyone who uses it? Mindfulness, clarity, independence, happiness, and life all flow naturally from the well that is us. We are well in health, dispersing so many with healing and caring, but we

need to learn to care for that room. Who knows, but we could overflow when we do?

With Stroke and Depression, Health Wellness Fitness

Your self-esteem takes a beating, and your overall fitness for health after having a stroke. Sadly, your family is hurting right alongside you. They have the responsibility of attempting to care for you in your recovery. You are now faced with two big obstacles as a stroke survivor, regaining your former physical ability and defeating the depression that is likely to follow.

According to a health-being exercise study, ten to twenty-seven percent of stroke survivors will experience major depression. Besides, 15 to 40% of people are expected to develop severe depression symptoms over the next two months. Sadly, it is likely to take up to one year for the depression to be treated satisfactorily.

There appears to be a correlation between the severity of the depression and the patient's loss of functionality. It's easy to get overwhelmed when a long recovery period looms ahead, and there's no assurance that the victim can recover full functioning. Behavioral and personality changes can be likely depending on the severity and location of the stroke. Such improvements will delay recovery.

There is a possibility that when the changes are accompanied by depression that could go unnoticed, the changes may be put down to being induced by the stroke. Not every survivor of a stroke has depression,

but a significant number do. If you know or care about someone who has recently had a stroke, bear in mind that they may not have been diagnosed with depression and that the onset of depression may occur or has already occurred without your knowledge. If any depression is handled rapidly, a person recovering from a stroke stands a greater chance of a faster recovery.

Following a stroke, numerous different signs of depression have been reported. For more than two weeks, someone who has undergone five or more of these symptoms is advised to seek medical attention from their general practitioner as soon as possible.

* An ongoing mood of sadness which may be persistent

* Easily irritated

* Crying excessively

* Consistent Chronic aches or pains that don't seem to respond to treatment

Many people suffering from major depression after a stroke has found that being treated for their depression with antidepressants has helped boost their overall fitness for health. This increase in their ability to cope has helped them make a faster recovery. Naturally, family members must keep physicians and therapists aware of any medical or behavioral changes that arise. These adjustments may be responsible for a medical interaction, or it may be something that changes with the patient's health, and it is important to determine the cause. Being mindful of all these possibilities and the fact that depression is likely to accompany a stroke will ensure that the best possible treatment for a stroke victim is given the best recovery chance.

CHAPTER 2:

IMPORTANCE OF THE NUTRITION HEALTH WELLNESSTRIANGLE IN OUR LIFE

In terms of nutritional health, life is not a matter of living and dying, unlike what most people think; it is not measured by total life and death. Rather, it is being measured around a health continuum, one on which death is on one end and good well-being, not just being alive, on the other. So, we can assume that the healthier one is, the further he is from death, by using the continuum of nutritional health well-being. The passing of time is immediately taken into account in this situation since one's health will usually begin to deteriorate at a certain age.

Even if health degradation is unavoidable as time passes (at least in fact, although not in theory), we can still do something about our health nutrition, fitness lifestyles, and activities to slow down the deterioration of health in a variety of ways - or rather, a variety of ways that must be incorporated. Proper physical activity, a balanced psychological outlook, and carefully designed nutrition are some of these nutrition health wellness enhancement strategies, with the latter being the subject of this report.

Why is it important for fitness, nutritional wellbeing, and longevity to have the right food? Our bodies are fed and preserved by a range of chemicals, mainly oxygen, hydrogen, carbon, and other essential elements such as

calcium, iron, and zinc. Both of these, excluding oxygen that can be absorbed through breathing, can only be taken by eating and drinking, or in other words, through feeding. Food is the cornerstone and corner of the health nutrition wellbeing triangle because these chemicals encourage and improve our minds and bodywork. Without adequate nutrition, the body lacks the energy it needs to carry out its activities, preventing proper physical exercise or wellness activity and, as a result, lowering health.

An individual without the proper nutrition required by the mind would not be capable of greater psychological processes on the psychological side, so the need for a healthy psychological disposition is also far from accomplished. In terms of one's nutritional health wellbeing, it is important to note that scientists still support the concept that the mind can overpower its design, particularly its consciousness. Although this is real, the value of adequate food consumption in raising our own nutrition health wellbeing triangle cannot be overstated.

Health Wellness Tips

It often seems difficult to follow through with even the most simple and well-known healthy behaviors in today's fast-paced world. But when it comes to incorporating the following lifestyle tips for fitness, everything is much better than nothing.

Balanced eating is the first one and one of the most important. On the other hand, who has the time or incentive to consume five or more fruits and vegetables every day? And if you're trying to keep an eye on your weight, the extra calories are hard to afford. So here's a suggestion: a banana for breakfast and a Ziploc bag of sweet and low-calorie baby carrots for an afternoon snack. Then, to make sure you're getting enough of your micronutrients, take a quick multivitamin/mineral supplement.

Second, and I'm sure you've heard it a thousand times before, proper water intake. Again, most people I know don't even come close to drinking the

required eight glasses a day. And if you only have 3 or 4 glasses a day, you'll be better off than if you don't have any. Making a drinking glass the first thing you do after crawling out of bed (or after your first bathroom trip!) is a simple thing to do. Now you've just got three to go for the rest of the day. Some people heat their water to get more fun out of it.

The third point, which has also been pounded into us, is having enough sleep. The time factor enters the picture once more (the lack of it). The majority of us do not get the recommended eight hours of sleep. But

a power nap and a little practice will help you get through the day. It can take a few tries to quiet your mind enough to fall asleep for 15 to 20 minutes, but once you've mastered it, it can be a lifesaver. When you're emotionally fading, it will help you get back on track and even reduce tension.

You will enjoy all of the benefits of healthy living without burning yourself out by attempting the often-unrealistic goals set for us to achieve optimal health by integrating a few basic health wellness tips into your everyday life. Something is as good as nothing!

Five Essential Wellness Secrets for Fitness

This time, I'm doing something different. Instead of the normal accident and neuromuscular dysfunction, I'm going to talk about health wellness. If you regularly workout and do yoga, are you contributing to your wellness? You are, without a doubt. What about supplementing your diet with vitamins and minerals? Without question. Some good health components remain healthy with regular exercises and maintain a balanced diet and nutrition. There are, however, five components of wellbeing.

The majority of people were already conscious of the value of exercise and a good diet. Rest is the third aspect of wellness. That is right. To relax. When you're intoxicated, passing out is not called rest. Believe me when I say that. I had a try, and it didn't succeed. Throughout the day, the body and mind experience several physical stresses and mental

stress. Before starting a new day, the cells of your body and mind need to recharge fully.

Have you ever met or worked with someone bitter, skeptical, and pessimistic? Unfortunately, many people see the world through a half-empty eye. The fourth aspect of health, I believe, is the most difficult to attain. You must continually train your mind and remind yourself to have a good mental attitude (PMA). Not quick, but it's doable. If I can develop a PMA, then you can, too.

There's going to be a moment when you forget PMA, and you're going to fall. You might be irritable and easy to get upset about something. You may come to regret what you've done or said. And that's perfect. All of us are people, and nobody is fine. Knowing what you did or said and not doing it in the future is the secret to PMA.

Let's think about exercise, diet, rest, and a healthy mental attitude before disclosing the last wellness aspect. Daily workouts keep you involved. You eat well and take supplements. You pass out; I mean, every night, you sleep soundly. You are confident and still look on the bright side. You still don't have any discomfort, stiffness, or other symptoms. Your blood pressure, blood sugar, and cholesterol levels are healthy. And twice a day, you wash and floss your teeth. You've got this health thing down, sweetheart. You're a superstar for wellbeing.

So, what else isn't there? How about getting your muscles, joints, and spine taken care of? You use your muscles, joints, and spine while you are involved.

Without them, you wouldn't be able to walk, run, ride your bike, do yoga or work out at the gym.

During everyday life, the muscles, joints, and spine undergo much physical pressure and stress. Exercises and other physical movements increase these mechanical stresses and stress. About why? And as you move, the muscles, joints, and spine move. Daily life, workouts, and poor postures cause micro-traumatic injuries to your muscles, joints, and spine, similar to the mechanical wear and tear of your car's engine and brakes. Why do you think people get more pressure, stiffness, and other muscle, joint, and spine issues.

when they grow older? Aches, pains, tightness, and stiffness become more persistent as the wear and tear wounds accumulate.

So, how do you keep your muscles, joints, and spine dried out mechanically? This is fast with chiropractic preventive care. It's no different than your car having a tune-up, or an oil change every day. And that's all right—all it's about having a positive mental outlook, kid. Preventive chiropractic therapy is the final component of wellbeing. Think about this before you roll your eyes.

Spinal and joint chiropractic improvements restore natural motion, which reduces mechanical wear and tear and increases mobility. Chiropractic soft tissue therapies minimize and avoid fibrosis scar tissue development in the muscles, decreasing muscle

strain and stress during exercise and other physical activities.

Let's be frank. I know that chiropractic is not for everyone, even with my optimistic attitude. Chiropractic treatment, whether for acute or preventative wellbeing, will make you feel better. When you receive chiropractic treatment, you'll easily understand why so many patients refer to chiropractors as "miracle workers."

Mental Wellbeing & Health Basics

Whether you're at the top of the planet, in a deep, suicidal funk, or floating peacefully down the middle of the road; achieving and sustaining mental wellbeing and wellness has five basics: a balanced diet, adequate sleep, regular exercise, sufficient medical treatment, and social-emotional relations.

A Healthful Diet

Eating the right amount of food increases brain activity and cognitive processes. Fresh fruits and vegetables, particularly deep red and orange and dark, leafy greens—provide abundant vitamins, minerals, and fiber that go a long way to fuel the body and mind. Foods high in omega-3 fatty acids

(including salmon, linseeds, walnuts, cauliflower, cabbage, broccoli, spinach, halibut, tofu, Brussels sprouts, green beans, scallops, fish, cod, and strawberries) improve brain function by enhancing sleep and concentration, decreasing the probability of Alzheimer's and depression, and lowering blood pressure and cholesterol, thereby reducing the risk of

stroke. In addition, drinking eight or more cups of water a day and an occasional glass of red wine keeps cells hydrated and adds antioxidants, respectively. The well-fed body facilitates the optimum functioning of the brain.

Adequate Sleep

Any insomniac can show that lack of sleep leads to muddled thinking, inefficient decision-making, irritability, and depression. When the brain cannot join the REM loop, and the body cannot release the day's accumulated stress, mental well-being and comprehension suffer. Human beings are designed to spend about one-third of every twenty-four hours sleeping. If you regularly get less than that, the reserves will be drained, and the body and brain function will suffer. On the other hand, if you sleep a lot more than the required 8 hours every night, lethargy will take over, and it becomes a struggle to get enough of the next basic requirement to maintain mental health and wellness: exercise.

Regular Exercise

You don't have to prepare for a marathon or ride a bike 50 miles a week to get enough exercise. Slowly walking for thirty minutes a day, five days a week, is a decent aim for most people and enough exercise to keep muscles toned, weight in control, and the circulatory system working properly, both of which support brain function and mental health. As long as you move your body and increase blood flow, every activity you enjoy is a healthy one. For others, it's going to be yoga; for others, kickboxing or ballet. It's

the point, Pass. Switch at least thirty minutes a day, five days a week.

Proper medical care

Annual check-ups and age-appropriate lab work and studies catch health issues before they become full-blown problems. And because all individuals have specific genetic profiles and predispositions, some people need to see a doctor regularly for chronic or severe conditions. An individual with diabetes must track various aspects of his or her health. An individual with rheumatoid arthritis must consult a doctor regularly. Those with brain disorders would do the same thing. Clinical depression, bipolar disorder, and schizophrenia fall under this category and should be managed for optimum health and rehabilitation.

Proper medical treatment keeps each of these people safe and well so that they can enjoy the pleasures of everyday community life. And that takes us to the very last of the basics: friendship.

Social-Emotional Connection

Relationships, or social-emotional connections, help health at all stages. People with strong and meaningful relationships, both personal and friendly, appear to be more physically involved. They get out more, engage in many physical and mental events, chat more, listen more, think more, touch more, care more. Their physical needs are more readily met, their emotional needs are discussed, their minds stimulated, and their spirits nurtured. The entire person is better linked to others in caring and appreciative relationships

Accept your condition with all this in mind. Do you do whatever you can to keep your body and mind healthy? Is your routine leading to mental health and well-being? Are you eating a balanced diet? Get enough sleep? Do you exercise regularly? Looking for proper medical care? And enjoying a good relationship? If you can answer "yes" to every question, Bravo! Keep it up, man. But if you find your routine lacking in one area or another, consider the above suggestions and start implementing   .

CHAPTER 3:

PERSONAL DEVELOPMENT
HEALTH & WELLNESS INSPIRATION

Do you feel like you're able to start taking better care of yourself? You may feel a little under the weather, searching for ways to bring about positive changes in your life. This is going to help.

There are many old sayings along the lines of doing to yourself what you'd expect people to do to you, what's going on, and what's going on.

My view is that first and foremost, we need to take good care of ourselves.

You're the most important thing in your life. Time! Period!

For a large part of what we teach, I work closely with **Personal Development to concentrate on being safe and fit. I also deal with the Rule of Attraction, which tells us** that what we think about is what we bring about and that our emotions also influence the stuff we bring into our lives. When you realize this, it makes too much sense to concentrate on your health and well-being before bringing in any other meaningful life improvements.

Your wellbeing and happiness are the secrets to having a more satisfying and happier life when you've got this part of your life to move on to the growth of another field of your life.

Think of the three terms Mind, Body, Spirit. Healthy Body, Healthy Mind, Healthy Spirit.

We do feel better about the whole when we feel safe. If you feel a little under the weather right now, I would highly recommend reading You Can Cure Your Life by Louise Hay. This is a great introduction to the influence of personal growth when it comes to fitness and wellness.

Have you ever heard of the three steps to fitness, wellness, and longevity? It is very necessary in today's world to have a balanced diet. But I'm not talking about a diet. I am referring to dietary supplements. Most of the people I interact with are taking a multi-vitamin, a healthy course of action. However, whenever I discuss the three stages, most people don't know what I'm talking about. Let me go over these three steps briefly.

The three steps are to detoxify your body, feed your body and retain your youth. Detoxifying the body is the first step towards a healthy approach to dietary supplements. Let's say, for example, that I have an apple, and I cut the apple in half. What's going to happen to the apple? The apple will soon turn brown when exposed to air or free radicals. Well, the same air that makes the apple brown can make our

machine rust on the inside. So, the first step is a strong antioxidant to keep our system running properly on the inside.

Phase two is to feed our bodies with a high-quality mineral supplement. Did you know the body needs 86 trace minerals a day to work properly? The sugar craving is the result of a mineral deficiency.

The third and final step is to retain your youth with a high-quality immune system supplement. Practicing a 3-step approach to health, wellbeing, and longevity will improve your vitality and sharpen your mind.

Taking dietary supplements is not a luxury; it is a requirement. In the past, much of our vitamins and minerals came directly from the food we consumed. However, due to the depletion of minerals in the soil from which the food is produced, we must supplement it. Much as a fish is as nutritious as the water in which it swims, the nature of our food is just as good as the soil in which it grows.

So, we need to learn how to complement science and nature in dietary supplements better. With new advances in science and nature, the standard of supplements has risen to a higher level. Keep away from synthetic vitamins and minerals that are mainly starchy and contain very few vitamin minerals.

Focus on herbal and herbal vitamins that work in the biochemistry of your body. The 3-step process of detoxifying your body, feeding your body, and preserving your youth along with a diet of living food for the living body will help to build a balanced approach to the overall health and well-being.

Health & Wellness Program Ideas

Health and wellness programs and facilities are designed to facilitate healthy lifestyle habits and reduce health care expenses. The emphasis is on avoiding disease and injury, improving wellness and efficiency, and lowering healthcare costs. A good health and wellness program supports employers by creating and sustaining a healthy, more efficient workforce and society. It helps workers by enhancing their physical and mental health.

Health and wellness services are designed to improve and encourage health and fitness. They are typically sold via the workplace, while insurance policies can be offered directly to their customers. The service allows the boss or plans to give you premium discounts, cash incentives, gym memberships, and many other forms of opportunity to join. Examples of wellness services include programs to help you avoid smoking, diabetes management programs, weight loss programs, and preventive health screening. Some

companies are providing discounts on your health insurance premium if you meet certain criteria. E.g.,

You're going through a series of steps, working out several days, following weight guidelines, and stopping smoking.

Good workers cost employers less. Studies have shown that workers who participated in services are less likely to leave and pursue additional jobs. Employees are sick less, health care expense savings, improved efficiency, higher morale, and employee pride are only a few of the advantages of health promotion and wellness services.

Johnson & Johnson initiated the software in 1995. Since then, workers who smoke have fallen by more than two-thirds. The number of people who have high blood pressure or are sedentary decreased by more than half. Well, it turns out that a systematic, carefully planned investment in the social, mental, and physical health of workers pays off. Johnson & Johnson reports that their wellness services have saved the organization $250 million in health care expenses over the last decade, with a return of $2.71 for every dollar invested between 2002 and 2008. I'm not that great at math, but I know it's a lot of money.

Wellness services have been used in the past as a nice benefit, not a requirement. Times have changed, and evidence indicates that both worker's and employers' bank accounts are successful. With tax credits and grants available under existing federal health care laws, businesses can use wellness services to reduce their huge cost of health care and have happier, more efficient workers. It's a win-win thing.

Any business or organization should have an expert who creates and implements a simple, thorough wellness program. Programs are designed to reduce health risks, enhance the quality of life, improve personal productivity, and support its bottom line. You can't enforce a program. It's got to be a business way of life. Health and wellness services are still a work in progress. I've read that Virgin Mobile has no chairs at all. Of course, you need to keep the meetings short and to the point. Encourage the use of the stairs if you've got them.

Some methods of supporting workers in health and fitness activities are as follows:

Give a discount on your insurance premium. Memberships (or discounts) to wellness clubs, have healthy snacks, have walking meetings, have a team contest, start a stretch break or two every day, have reward gift cards. Put on fun posters with wellness ideas all over the office to keep a healthy lifestyle at the forefront. Give apple stress balls to encourage healthy snacks. Give discounts on activity trackers and set unique targets. Using the resistance bands to facilitate exercise. Provide health journals to workers to keep track of progress on their objectives. Celebrate the Health & Wellness Day with enjoyable games and play. Get the business walk 10K and provide the FM radios. Compile a safe company cookbook or provide each employee with one that has already been printed. If you want a very fun, competitive price, have a team challenge (a team that loses the most weight, inches, or exercises the most) with a nice big reward for the winning team. Perhaps the reward could be a holiday or a night out in a limo area.

Once you get started, you'll find employees who inspire each other and expand to friends and family outside your business.

CHAPTER 4:

HEALTH, WELLNESS, AND BALANCE AFTER 50

Good health, what does it mean? ... It means different things in your life at different times. You're expected to have a solid, safe body in your 20's. By the age of 30, you begin to see that you can't take anything for granted and that you can pay a little more attention to your diet and how much exercise you get. Your 40's are beginning to show the results of past neglect. Baking in the sun to get the golden tan in your teens and the twenties show up in the fine lines that accentuate your eyes or probably skin cancer.

By the time you turn 50, you actively try to turn back the clock. Your energy might be better spent repurposing your life to establish a balance between your Body, Mind, and Spirit. This alone will prepare you for the years to come in a way that will bring both optimal health and ultimate happiness.

Our body must be kept in good repair because we take it with us into our old age. We feel best when we pursue a lifestyle that focuses on good health based on disease prevention. We know that eating a diet rich in fruits and vegetables is necessary for healthy living and regular exercise. Haven't you been doing a great job with this? Making changes doesn't have to be difficult but works better with a consistent effort. The wisdom of eating an apple a day has proven true, so start with that. Did you know walking just 10 minutes

a day can boost your energy level and help your joints work smoother? Getting adequate relaxation is vital for the care of your whole self. Do you sleep soundly? Sleep is recuperative. Constant sleep deprivation predisposes you to several health problems. If you are having trouble sleeping at night, increasing your daily exercise may help. Taking a simple 15-minute nap can help you get through your day in addition to recharging your internal healing system. Our bodies are wonderful machines, but we need to keep them well oiled by paying attention to daily maintenance, thus keeping them optimal.

Improving your mental state is a lifelong challenge. Finding new outlets for using your gifts in one of the many volunteer opportunities that abound keeps your mind sharp while widening your worldly perspective of being in touch with and serve others. Serving others deepens our sense of gratitude which strengthens balance.

Have you lost contact with who you are right now? Take time out every day to spend some quality time alone. Rediscover what is energizing you. Do you want to paint? Just do that. Do you want to sing? Join the nearest chorus. Look deep in your heart to see what makes you live. Take steps to do those things.

For many, the protection of the soul is the anchor of equilibrium and good overall health. Having strong beliefs and principles will improve any aspect of well-being. Belief in a higher force, whatever you call it, will give you the courage to survive and resolve many challenges in your life. Spirituality is key to health and allows you to survive when you feel the lowest and most helpless. How are you going to feed your spirit? Again, the secret is simplicity. Walk-in early morning light is energizing and helps you keep in step with your body's circadian rhythm. Fill your home with music or work of art that speaks to your soul. A cup of tea and a peaceful moment will work well to get you back in touch with your inner wisdom. Spending daily time in prayer or meditation contributes to a deeper understanding of life.

Body, mind, and spirit; all work together. Holding your life in order is the greatest gift you can offer yourself when you get older. You can note subtle

improvements in your attitude, outlook, and energy level over time as you become the best you can be after 50.

Women's Health & Wellness

As a woman, you need to educate yourself about every aspect of women's health since it includes a wide range from general health to a narrower emphasis on reproductive health. Women's wellbeing is a huge concern, from pregnancy to infection to infertility.

When it comes to wellbeing, men and women experience and respond differently to different circumstances. Both ought to participate in preventive measures as this increases their quality of life.

The topic of women's health is rising. Many details about this subject can make it a little bit complicated, but you'll find that the basics stay the same as you're going through it.

There are also many items out there to help women tackle different health problems, but you should still be educated on what you are taking. The internet is a perfect way to do this. Several forums and groups discuss the items they have used and the benefits or disadvantages they have faced when taking them.

Like anything else, it's all about having the right facts. But you can need to dig deep and double-check the numerous official references.

As we all know, when it comes to your wellbeing, what you eat is significant. Shockingly, some of the essential ingredients needed to have a balanced diet are often not in short supply in the food we consume every day.

The good news is that nutritious foods are readily available in your local grocery store, but you will need to make extra efforts to find them. It's interesting how nutrient-robbing foods seem to be more prevalent than balanced foods.

Women have many health problems to contend with, for example, breast cancer. It's really necessary as a woman that you do daily mammograms as a preventive measure. Exercise is necessary, as normal. It is also important that you cultivate healthy habits, such as drinking plenty of water, consuming fresh food such as fruit and vegetables, and maintaining a balanced diet.

Know that prevention is often easier than treatment. Daily exercise and healthy eating habits are going to do a lot to boost your lifestyle and self-image. It can also help with the mental health and general life outlook, and, along with this, daily exercise has been shown to reduce the severity of menstrual cramps.

Sleep is finally another main aspect of wellbeing. Sleep deprivation is not good for you, and several studies report on various health problems that may occur due to lack of sleep. In conclusion, eat well, exercise, and get regular check-ups for optimum wellbeing.

Laughter's Wellbeing Wellness Advantages

When was the last time you had a good belly to laugh at? The health benefits of laughter are too many to be laughed at. A strong intestine-buster strengthens the diaphragm and abdominal muscles. It enhances healthy blood flow, decreases serum cortisol (stress hormone) levels, activates endorphins (euphoric hormones), increases the pain threshold, and improves the immune system. Humor and laughter were uniquely human. Laughter cultivates a more relaxed social environment and produces an overall sense of well-being. So, lighten up and chuckle a bit, making life too short to be sad. Here are some tips to improve your humor:

View life from another perspective: Keep your life exciting. Find new ways to do stuff that you do every day, or try something you've never done before.

Express instead of impression: Impression is always shallow and selfish, whereas speech is advantageous to all concerned.

You're going to find this more of an icebreaker while laughing at someone else is an icebreaker.

Find a funny role model here: Read or listen to the jokes or comedians you find amusing. Ask yourself, what makes this guy so funny? Hang out with funny friends who make you laugh, and eventually... Plan for leisure and have some fun with you. You can visit a comedy club, get together with funny friends, sit at home and watch a funny show or movie. Oh, that's good medicine now.

Fake It: studies have shown positive results, whether a smile is true or false, and the same goes for laughter. You're still going to get the health benefits listed above, even if you fake-laugh.

CHAPTER 5:

A LIFE IN BALANCE

Relaxation and even mediation are more important than ever in the turmoil that affects us in our lives. It is an established reality that people who have been given or are demanding adequate downtime in their world are more often happier, healthier, and much less depressed.

It's not always possible to monitor the work or business climate, or anyone can afford to visit an expensive spa once or twice a week, which is why there's a growing demand for home spas. There are a lot of ways to find comfort and balance at home. They can be both large and small, and they can vary in price.

Swim Spas are the perfect way to carry the feeling of relaxation to your home without the need for membership, public baths, or costly treatments. A warm pool in your backyard for both fun and health; treatment pools can be built with very little square footage needed, yet the benefits can be practically unlimited. Your oasis is open 24 hours a day in the safety of your yard. Maintenance can be relatively simple, and most packages may provide ongoing support. There's not little standing between you and your home spa or relaxing area when you look closely.

Our mental, physical and emotional health, and wellbeing cannot be underestimated, particularly in today's challenging world. A swimming pool, therapy pool, or sauna can be just what you need to keep your life in order because life is easier if it's balanced.

The secret to Health & Wellness Is Not Secret.

You saw the make-up of a human cell. Whether it's a type of cancer, obesity, skin disorders, sleep disorders, bone disorders, heart disease, the fundamental reality is that all health and wellness issues are primarily caused by what you eat, something you can't manage, a lack of exercise, plain and simple. If the truth is said, you're what you're eating.

When you begin to understand why the body, with its complex system, is mainly made up of water, proteins, amino acids, etc., and the function of any part of the body, such as the primary purpose of the colon, which is to remove fluids and nutrients from solid food for distribution, then you have to believe that nature plays a crucial role in our well-being, as it was meant and will always be.

So, without having to give you a hint as to the link between the earth's water source, the piles of soil foliage and the tree system, and the human body (DNA-RNA), remember that there is a fine balancing act between eating naturally and your wellbeing, no matter what your age and illnesses are!

Granted, it is not always possible to adhere to Mother Nature's natural properties in a hectic modern society. At the very least, though, one should make every effort to give the body what it needs by other types of natural products, such as omega-3sm, for those who do not eat fish regularly, as an example, to combat the toxins that come into your body system every day.

In retrospect, if you are searching for alternative therapies for cancer, breast cancer, prostate cancer, liver cancer, bowel cancer, lung cancer, and other diseases, note that most cancers are age-related. That is, the older you get, the more vulnerable you become to contracting cancer and other diseases for

a variety of reasons, but more importantly, because of a weakening and deteriorating a neglected immune system that has been continually exploited and bombed by free radicals (outside elements)! Your immune system must be restored to its natural battle capabilities by raising the amount of glutathione.

The secret of alternatives is no secret at all. You must return to the properties of nature to preserve the natural balance in your cells, which only nature (fruits, vegetables, fish) can provide, and in the meantime, increase your glutathione levels at all costs.

CHAPTER 6:

HEALTH & WELLNESS COACHING TIPS

Good habits and adequate nutrition are what we're trying to do, but many of us in this department are getting low. Improved wellbeing, which seems to be never-ending at times but possible, is what we would like to achieve. Our bodies are out of control and very complicated, so we're looking for wellness to get more energy. Your vitality is most likely to be there, and it just needs to be restored.

Glutathione is the body's most potent antioxidant and is more powerful than when vitamins C and E are consumed. And for those of you who are not acquainted with Glutathione, it is tripeptide (three proteins in one molecule); very important to cell function. It fights inflammation, increases stamina, enhances focus, and strengthens the immune system, to name a few of its benefits! When we reach our twenties, our Glutathione supply decreases from 10% to 15% in our bodies every ten years. This decreases our energy levels, damages our immune system, and much more.

Our resources, our healthy organs, and our skin need healthy cells. Today, if you want to add antioxidants to your diet, that's great. It's a great way to help your wellbeing, but Glutathione is a natural antioxidant provided by our bodies that is more important for protecting healthy cells.

Age is not always the guilty party when we lament stuff that we use to do but can no longer do. Stress, accidents, illnesses, and vigorous exercise, not to mention airborne toxins, are just some of the factors that substantially reduce or reduce Glutathione levels.

You want to live your life with Max! You have to fend off all the damaging things that affect your bodies to do that. Increased stamina, a powerful immune system, and high athletic efficiency are the way forward!

1. What is coaching?

Coaching is an evolving service profession focused on sport, business, spirituality, psychology, and organizational growth. It's about passionate people like you who want to get something out of their personal and business lives. A coach will help you set bigger, more fulfilling goals, build a plan to achieve them, and encourage the process, not unlike getting a personal trainer or athletic coach, transformational, except in a business and personal sense. Achieving goals is something that comes easier as a product of a coaching relationship.

2. Why is coaching working?

Coaching works when two variables are present: 1) the individual is eager to improve, and 2) there is a difference between where they are now and where they want to be.

Good coaching clients know the importance of sharing ideas with someone who knows them and is subjective enough to want a lot for them but reasonable enough not to be biassed or self-serving. Talking about choices with someone who can listen to them is always enough to be very

straightforward.

Coaching works with three specific features:

Synergy: Customer and coach become a team that works on the client's expectations and desires and does more than the client can do independently.

Structure: Coaching will provide transparency, inspire the client to take more initiative, think more, and get the job done.

Expertise: In addition to coaching skills, each coach may also have the advanced expertise to help clients make better choices, set the right goals, learn new communication skills and restructure their personal and professional lives for optimal contentment efficiency.

3. Where are you going to start with a coach?

Many coaches begin with a special client meeting or call to get to know each other. The coach wants to learn about the client's ambitions, desires, and challenges. The client needs to be familiar with the coach. At this meeting, both parties will draw up a list of priorities and a game plan to achieve these objectives.

4. How are coaching sessions going to work?

Coaching is generally performed on the phone. In addition to frequent, daily contact, it is easy to remain in a "coaching relationship" as the client can call from their office, home, car, or hotel. The coached person completes the coaching call plan form before each call, outlining the current challenges and the progress they have made since the last call. Most people are coached two hours a month, in either four 30-minute sessions, three 40-minute sessions, or two one-hour sessions.

The client shall decide the focus of each call. The coach allows them to see their challenges or problems from various viewpoints, helping them find new solutions. A coach can better educate clients by offering insight into the client's roadblocks' progress and helping them prepare to break through those blocks and celebrate the wins. There is also "fieldwork" where the client has a formula, a different insight, or a challenge to try something in a new way.

5. What happens when you enter into a deal with a coach?

You're taking yourself and what you want more seriously.

You automatically take more successful and concentrated action.

You're going to stop putting up with stuff that's going to get in your way.

You build momentum to accomplish more, be more balanced, and develop more effective management skills.

You have laid out personal goals that are transparent, and that fulfill your needs.

You recognize and remove obstacles that impede the achievement of your goals.

You communicate more responsibly about what you need and want from others.

6. How can a doctor be a coach, too?

Health and Wellness Coaching provides an atmosphere where participants can share the independence from judgment and demands that physicians and patients currently have in our traditional health care system. It's safe to challenge, appear insecure, observe, investigate, experiment, learn, and alter the coaching climate. This trust factor encourages the client to use the 'Doctor Coach' (or Health and Wellness Coach) to strengthen their health and well-being with confidence and anticipation that facilitates their progress.

Your Health and Wellness Coach will direct and educate you in ways that will help you accomplish your life goals, teach you how to raise your spirit, and nurture your soul. The achievement of these incredible heights involves a special coach/client relationship.

The Ten Commandments to Get True Health & Wellness

1. You will know how much food and nutrition you eat daily.

So often, people ingest unconsciously. By first learning what you need and then adding those things to your regular diet, you'll start developing a balanced outline. Knowing how much food you need every day will make you budget your intake more balanced. You need to consider your calorie flip point, which burns all the calories you eat, to keep your weight safe. You're going to flip because you eat more calories than you consume. You have to be past the flip stage to lose more weight if you have to flip 500 calories a day to lose ONE pound a week.

2. Add fruit and vegetables.

Nutrition is important for good health. If you don't plan fruit and vegetables in your diet, you probably won't eat them. They are not shelf-stable and are also not pre-packaged. In this comfort culture, nutritious foods are more of a challenge to eat. Eat a wide range of foods and colors since each color offers various types of nutritional benefits. Make your target of eating at least three "colors" a day.

3. Minimize and, where possible, eliminate highly processed foods containing artificial ingredients and additives.

It's a daunting but necessary part of every wellness plan. The more processed foods you eat, the more complicated your path to health and wellness would be. Try to make the Majority of your diet based on whole or natural foods. Some foods have not been modified or refined. Things like fresh or frozen fruit and vegetables, eggs, lean meats, and other natural, uncooked foods.

4. You shall drink water all day long.

A minimum of eight oz. Glasses per day. Water is important for life. For your body to work at its best, you need to maintain hydration as oil is in the engine, water in your body. To make your bodywork as it was made, you need to drink water every day.

5. You shall pass your body every day.

A sustained movement of at least 20 minutes per day is recommended. It would be best if you kept going to remain safe. Not only one kind of action, but a lot. The big three are Cardiopulmonary—gets a high heart rate, Strength Training—tunes the muscles and strengthens the bones, and Stretching/Range of Motion—keeps the body relaxed and healthy.

6. You're going to have a good night's sleep.

Sleep is of utmost importance to good health. At night, the body restores itself to a cellular level. You will perform at a sub-par level without sufficient rest. It's necessary to keep the mind quiet. Enable yourself to have the gift of rest.

7. You shall pursue self-enrichment regularly.

Spending time to invest in yourself is important for achieving peace in mind, body, and spirit. Build a habit of learning new things and ways of expressing yourself. Participation in an artistic outlet encourages well-being. This keeps your mind sharp and improves your mental and spiritual health. Look for uplifting and inspiring content to read or watch daily.

8. You are not going to be pessimistic.

Negative behaviors do not lead to good health. What you think and talk about has a direct impact on your well-being. Complaints, rumors, and feelings of inability will contribute to more of the same. Retrain your mind in all aspects to search for the positive. This change in attitude can increase endorphins.

9. You practice stress relief regularly.

Stress is a major risk factor for all types of disease. It's important to learn ways to relax and unwind. It's smart to do that every day. Before you understand how to control your tension, you can not improve your overall health and wellbeing.

10. Engage in the prevention and screening of health services.

Ignorance is no paradise! Not knowing about a health condition doesn't make it go away. Early detection and prevention can be the best protection against life-threatening conditions. The bottom line is, know your health statistics, have your annual scans, and see your doctor regularly as driven by your age and condition.

CHAPTER 7:

COMPARTMENTALIZE

Separate into distinct sections is what the term "compartmentalize" means. I am fascinated by the fact that there is the word "mental" in the word. It highlights, for me, the need to mentally isolate what we do. Separating tasks and performing them one at a time is one of the tricks I'm learning. That is difficult for me as a recovering multitasker, but I am starting to see the advantages of doing one thing at a time.

I recall being told that two cognitive tasks are hard to do at one time. As a conscious intellectual function, cognitive activity is defined. While I've always prided myself on being able to do two or three tasks at once, I'm starting to realize that my focus is split when I multitask, and I'm not producing the quality work I'd like. I have found that doing more than one thing sometimes takes longer because my focus is divided.

Classifying and focusing on one thing at a time is the key to getting things done and getting them done well.

I am splitting my day into tasks now. I make a plan of what I'll do from hour to hour. I split my day down into tasks instead of beginning the day with a list of things to do and assuming that I can focus on it as I go along. I'm going to spend an hour on Project A, 15 minutes making phone calls, and another

block of e-mail time. I will potentially get more done quicker with fewer errors and less stress by compartmentalizing my day. It all boils down to concentration.

I recall beginning a project in the morning and getting it finished by the end of the day. I let myself get sidetracked by all of the other stuff that needed my attention. Now I understand that if I concentrate on one task, I can complete it and move on to the next. This is not to say that it is easy because life does not always fit neatly into neat compartments. On the other hand, creating this structure makes it easier to deal with the unpredictable events that life throws my way.

With compartmentalization, the trick is to figure out what works best for you. It works better for me to plan my time in one-hour increments. If it does not take an hour for the project I am working on, I have generated free time to do something else or begin the next project. I've also learned to be adaptable and predict the unexpected. Just for that chance, I also add in extra time. It can seem to be quite formal, but there is a great deal of flexibility in the structure. I concentrate on getting one thing done at a time instead of trying to do it all at once, and I achieve more by the end of the day - and stop feeling scattered or as depressed as I once did.

Shutting Down

Imagine that your mind is under the influence of an alien. That's how fear works, after all. It regulates the functions of your brain's neurotransmitters. But by behavioral learning, this sort of anxiety disorder may be understood.

Anxiety may be a brain problem since the human brain is the commander of all human activities, and anxiety appears to take hold. Anxiety affects people in various ways. Some are shut down, while others become too busy all of a sudden.

Here's an example: George suffers from anxiety and mental fatigue. When his anxiety isn't serious, he will carry on with his everyday activities, but only

to a certain degree. He can normally solve several problems at once. But in a state of fear, he can only concentrate on one problem at a time. And his personal life must have nothing to do with the problem. In other words, since they are tasks that do not require his analysis or preference, George will focus on completing his office tasks. When he gets home, however, all of the official issues have become his issues, such as paying bills, getting food, caring for his family, the color of the curtains, the furniture arrangement, and so on, all of which require his decision, and he unexpectedly shuts down. Even though those aren't significant problems that don't take much consideration, George can't process them when he's nervous. And if he's pressured to make decisions on those topics, he erupts in laughter. George begins crying, pacing, heavy breathing, feeling dizzy and out of control later on.

In this case, the only approach is to make a list of his problems on a paper sheet. Then, one by one and one at a time, he will deal with them.

How do you know?

They automatically think of physical fitness when most people think of health. Some assume that all a person wants to be healthy is to ensure the body is physically healthy. Although being physically active can improve a person's mental health, many people suffer from poor mental health despite being physically fit. The truth is that an individual's mental health is just as important as a person's physical health. Both are important for a person's happiness and physical well-being. Think of what other individuals are like when they have poor mental health? Consequently, their bodies tend to suffer, whether by gaining extra weight or having a crippling addiction; both can lead to poor physical health.

If you want to stop depression, you need to take care of your mental health. If, however, one feels that they suffer from some depression and that most days they feel unhappy or sad, people may do some things to boost their mood and mental health. Having enough sleep is the first. The fact that the average person in North America does not get enough sleep cannot be overstated. Sleep deprivation can cause exhaustion and emotional outbursts.

It is also important that a person eats healthily. If the body doesn't get the right nutrients or vitamins, it can adversely affect a person's mental health because it lacks what it needs. Exercising can also help with a person's mental health and mood. Changing the routine or going out more with friends can also help change the mood a long way.

However, some people have a hard time changing their attitudes and mental wellbeing, and the ideas above don't seem to improve. It could be that certain issues from the past cause depression, it could be an inherited condition, or it could be that for so long, the person has been depressed that they don't know how to act otherwise. If all of these conditions are the case, having an online therapist might be a smart idea. Go online, perform a quick search, and then contact an online therapist who offers their services. Online therapy is becoming more common these days because it is easy and helps people get assistance without leaving their homes. The majority of people tend to meet with online counselors from the convenience of their own homes. To decide what may cause their depression, an online therapist will quickly work with the patient and help them get out of their depression. Many people who have sought online therapy for depression have found it beneficial and have changed their lives as a result. Anyone who feels depressed and isn't sure how to get out should seek support from an online counselor.

Being in denial

In denial, we're all. We'd barely make it through the day if we were afraid that we or someone we care for could die today. Life is unpredictable, and denial helps us deal with what we need to live and concentrate on. Denial, on the other hand, leads us to disregard issues for which there are remedies or to dismiss feelings and desires that, if addressed, will change our lives. Unfortunately, you won't know it if you're in denial.

Denial Forms and Degrees

Denial has been dubbed the symbol of addiction when it comes to codependency. This refers not only to addicts to drugs (including alcohol)

but also to their friends and family members. Abuse and other forms of addiction also contribute to this theory. We may use denial to various degrees.

• Denial that the problem, symptom, feeling, or need exists in the first degree.

• Second degree: mitigating or rationalizing the situation.

• Admitting it but ignoring the implications is the third degree.

Fourth degree: Unable to request assistance.

Consequently, denial doesn't always indicate that we don't see a problem; instead, we can rationalize, justify, or diminish its relevance or impact on us. Forgetting, outright misleading, or contradicting the truth due to self-deception are other forms of denial. Deeper still, things that are too difficult to recall or to think about can be repressed.

Reasons for Denial

Denial is a defensive mechanism that aids us. We use denial for many purposes, including avoiding physical or emotional discomfort, anxiety, guilt, or conflict. It's the first defense we learned as a child. I thought it was funny when, though the evidence was smeared all over his lips, my four-year-old son vigorously denied eating any chocolate ice cream. He had lied for the sake of self-preservation and fear of retribution. Denial is adaptive because it helps us cope with challenging feelings, such as in the initial stages of grief after a loved one's loss, particularly if there is sudden separation or death. Denial helps our body-mind to respond more gradually to the shock.

If we deny warning signs of a treatable disease or problem out of fear, it's not adaptive. Out of fear, many women postpone having mammograms or biopsies, while early detection leads to greater cancer care progress. We may deny that we lump by applying the different degrees above; next, rationalize that it's possibly a cyst; third, accept that it may or is cancer, but deny that it could lead to death; or admit all of the above and yet be reluctant to receive treatment.

Another big source of denial is internal competition. Children often, out of pain, suppress memories of violence because they depend on their parents, love them, and avoid leaving home. Young children have idealized parents. It's easier to forget, rationalize, or make excuses than to face the unthinkable fact that my mother or father is cruel or crazy. Instead, they point the finger in their direction.

We reject the facts as adults when it may mean that we should take action that we don't want to take. We do not look at how much debt we have accrued because it would force us to decrease our spending or living standards, causing internal tension. Since facing the truth requires her to face not only the pain of adultery, embarrassment, and loss but also the likelihood of divorce. This woman notices facts from which she can conclude that her husband is cheating could rationalize and offer other explanations for the evidence. Since he'd have to deal with his marijuana addiction if he didn't look the other way when his child got high, an addicted parent could look the other way when his child gets high.

Denial is a popular "merry-go-round" for spouses of addicts or abusers. Addicts and abusers may be caring and even accountable and pledge to avoid their use or misuse of drugs, but it comes back quickly, breaking trust and promises. Since the partner loves them, may deny their own needs and worth, and is afraid of breaking the relationship, apologies and commitments are made and believed once more.

Another factor we dismiss issues is that we are used to them. We grew up with them and never knew something was wrong. Consequently, if we were emotionally exploited as children, we would not consider our spouse's mistreatment to be abuse. We could not notice or prevent our child from being incested if we were molested. This is referred to as a first-degree denial. Alternatively, we can agree that our partner is verbally abusive but downplay or rationalize it. Even though her husband was physically abusive, one woman told me she knew he loved her. Third-degree denial is encountered by most abuse victims, meaning they do not understand the negative effect

the abuse has on them - sometimes leading to PTSD long after leaving the abuser. They'd be more likely to seek help if they faced the facts.

Codependents, as described in my novel, Conquering Shame, and Codependency, have internalized shame from childhood. Shame is a highly painful emotion. Most individuals, including myself, have not known for many years how much shame drives their lives, even though they believe their self-esteem is pretty good. Usually, codependents often deny the needs and feelings of "shame-bonded" because they have neglected or shamed those needs and feelings. They may not be conscious of a feeling of guilt, such as fear or anger; they may diminish or rationalize it, or they may not be aware of how much it affects them. A big explanation for codependents to stay dissatisfied in relationships is the denial of needs. They reject problems and deny that their needs are not being addressed. They don't know that that's the case. They will feel bad if they do and lack the confidence to ask for what they need or know how to meet their needs. A big part of healing is learning to recognize and communicate our emotions and desires, and it is important for well-being and fulfilling relationships.

How to figure out if you're in denial

You may be unsure how to say whether you're delusory. Signs are there. Some of them have already been listed, such as rationalization, making excuses, forgetting, and minimization. Do your partner's actions affect his or her work, family, and social responsibilities, or your relationship if you're in a relationship with a drug user or drinker? There are more here. You do:

1. Consider how you would like things to be in your relationship.

2. Think to yourself

3. Do you doubt or deny your emotions?

4. Believe in repeated promises that are broken?

5. Is it possible to keep embarrassing parts of your relationship hidden?

6. Do you expect things to get better when something happens (such as a holiday, a change, or getting married)?

7. Make compromises and placate, hoping someone else can change that?

8. Does your partner feel resentful or used?

9. Have you spent years hoping that your relationship will improve or that anyone will change?

10. Walk on eggshells, worry about your partner's whereabouts, or fear talking about issues?

Learn more about codependency and enter a 12-Step program if you responded yes to all of these questions. By pointing out your defenses, challenging inconsistencies between your thoughts and reality, identifying denied emotions and desires, and helping you confront your fears and inner conflicts and make improvements, a competent therapist will aid your recovery. Codependency and addiction, like any disease, worsens without medication, but there is hope, and people will heal and live happier, more satisfying lives.

How to stay mentally well.

You will discover different editorials, materials, strategies, and methods every time you search for "how to remain mentally active," which are far too difficult to follow and not easy to bear in mind. You won't remember all the steps you need to take for a specific exercise until you've done reading the file. I've read many editorials, and the bulk of them include routine physical activities, certain nutritional diets, and complicated psychological games.

If anyone can find the time and commitment to implement these suggestions, it's awesome. However, bear in mind that most people are too preoccupied with work and family responsibilities to participate. They could barely find time for difficult brain games to train. Even if they are at risk of a

heart attack, some people refuse to adopt a certain diet. So, here are a few easy tips for keeping your mind engaged.

Put the hand on the opposite side of the table into play. It would be best if you turned your cursor to the other side of your hand to do that. By doing this, you stimulate the bond between the brain's two hemispheres. Clicking the mouse with the opposite hand is something that can quickly incorporate into your everyday routine.

If you are among those who spend a lot of time in front of the PC, it would be particularly easy to do. During the first few days, you might feel strange, and at first, you may feel like stepping back, but keep trying. Do not quickly give up. After a short time of adaptation, you'll be able to handle the programs with both hands.

Using the non-dominant side, you should try to perform as many tasks as possible, but others may become even heavier after a long time.

Play games that make you think. To get your mind in good shape, you don't need to solve any complicated math issues. Playing hidden object games or tasks as basic as crosswords or Sudoku can have the requisite effect on improving your brain's efficiency.

Play video games or board games along with other people when possible; you can remain socially involved and mentally engaged by doing so. Competing while playing a time-limited game can push you to concentrate more quickly and process data.

The regularity of playing this kind of game is an essential rule that you must consider. Try to integrate this brain conditioning into your everyday routine. And if you have a full day of tasks, you can always spend a few minutes doing this workout.

Do not forget that the mind is a muscle that requires exercise daily. It won't perform very well if you don't keep it in shape. So, what are you going to wait for? Start to practice these quick exercises.

Self-care

To you, what does self-care mean? " When you hear the words "self-care," what comes to mind? To different individuals, it can mean a lot of different things. Some of the answers I had when I asked individuals what it means to them include· Taking time off for me· Eating healthy· Eating healthy· Eating healthy· Eating healthy· Exercising· Getting a great massage!

To me, self-care involves simply looking after your entire self, not because you have to, but because you want to, because it feels good to do so, and because you enjoy taking care of your own as well as others' needs, and it is such an important thing to do for yourself. We can only give to others when we have enough inside ourselves to give. Allow yourself to become exhausted, tired, dehydrated, nutritionally deficient, emotionally exhausted, and physically exhausted. You can not enjoy life or be there for the important people in your life.

By caring for yourself properly, you relieve stress in your own life. You increase satisfaction, grow a balanced mind and body, and make life happier. Self-care has also helped minimize burnout, but it shows that you are a respected person, most importantly. That your needs are just as important as anyone else's and that taking care of yourself isn't selfish or self-indulgent; it's simply a form of self-respect.

There's a distinction between consuming fast food only because, opposed to making yourself a tasty and healthy meal, you're hungry and need a quick fix. Quick food satisfies your appetite, but a healthy meal satisfies your whole self, including your hunger, as well as your body and mind. You can either take a short shower to clean up or relax in a warm bath with Epsom Salts and essential oils. Again, all of these accomplish the purpose of getting clean; however, the bath takes care of you all - allowing you to relax, unwind, have time off, and get clean, instead of the rush that will give you a quick rinse off in the tub.

Ladies will also tell me that they don't do much self-care, either because it's too expensive or because they don't have time. Some self-care habits can potentially be costly, but you can do plenty of other things as well. Facials, massages, manicures, retreats, yoga lessons, and other spa treatments may all be great ways to pamper yourself, but they all come at a cost. For these types of transactions, you should set aside a small sum of money per week and reward yourself once a quarter, for example. These same luxuries can be had for a fraction of the price at home, and you'll always feel amazing afterward.

Yes, self-care acts aren't always possible regularly - we don't all have time to soak in the tub for an hour every day. Nevertheless, there are many self-care practices that you may incorporate that can easily become routines in your life and other activities that you may want to prepare on a weekly or fortnightly basis in time for.

1 Using a slice of lemon in hot water instead of coffee in the morning

2 Give yourself a manicure and hand massage

Taking a nap is number three on the chart.

4 Drawing, painting, making, and so on.

5 Listen to some songs

6 Meditate by meditating

7 Taking a stroll on the beach (or your other favorite spot) 8 Getting a foam roller and massaging your aching muscles

9 Getting workout

10 Creating a nutritious and balanced meal

11 Reading

12 Begin gathering compliments in a jar. Please write down something good anyone says to or about you and put it in your compliments jar. Re-read all the wonderful things people say about you now and then.

13 Stretch your body, or better yet, find a yoga workout on YouTube and give it a decent workout.

14 Get some fresh air.

15 Take a dip

16 Take it easy. Slow down your speed, put your phone away, and try to find five beautiful things in your surroundings.

17 Keep a record of thanks and milestones. Write five things you're thankful for every day and something you're proud of doing on that day

18 Give yourself a facial

Stuff like a regular doctor, dentist, option appointments, for instance, are other self-care facets. Is there a small health condition that has plagued you, but you never seem to get around to having the doctor's appointment? If it was a member of your child or family, would you make sure they were checked out?

When you become distracted, exhausted, or depressed, self-care is always the first thing to be overlooked, and yet it is the very thing you should turn to at these moments. Many people think of self-care as a reward or treat, but if you start integrating it into your daily and weekly routines, you'll see big changes in your life. If you feel overwhelmed or have forgotten what self-care feels like, take some time today to pick out a few things that you can do every day that only take care of you, and then pick out another activity you can do every week, maybe longer.

CHAPTER 8:

WELLBEING AND SOLUTIONS

It is always necessary to take care of oneself by applying all the principles of good health. Daily check-ups, a good diet, and safe living make it possible to stay on top of one's health in a cautious yet rational manner. Sometimes one is too obsessed with health problems and caught up in a loop of health concerns. One health problem is reconciled when another shows up immediately to take its place. After a while, these concerns become all-encompassing and stressful.

Eventually, the person understands that this cycle of health anxieties has compromised their quality of life. This intrusive aspect of anxiety must be resolved by the dark cloud, which is still looming over everyday life. One starts by deciding why this occurs, what function it serves, and how this activity can be disrupted.

Reason for Anxiety in Health

Health concerns serve a reason, and this purpose is not difficult to detect if one looks closely into this pattern of actions. Sometimes this pattern involves distracting the brain from real feelings that the person finds difficult to handle.

Many feelings are so overwhelming, such as rage, sadness, or fear, that the brain is searching for ways to distract. Health concerns suit the bill, and when you're deeply worried about your health, there's no place to discuss your troubling emotions.

Health is preoccupied with every other thinking, and this works. This is the ideal diversion from disquieting feelings. When one worry is reconciled, another takes the place of veiling undisguised emotion. Every health issue has a strong reason, as it hides a truly disturbing emotion that is far more difficult to confront in the long run.

Solution-Recognition and acknowledgment of the Health Anxiety habit, one concern immediately replacing the other in a visible loop that never ends. Knowledge of this cycle is often the first step towards reconciling the problem.

- It is difficult to decide whether this health condition is a real medical issue by consulting one's primary physician and ruling out a particular physical cause. Often rule out a physical trigger before thinking that it is just anxiety about wellbeing.

- Noting that these health issues are settled when you become deeply involved in another subject or get into a new relationship, work, or cause.

- Identify your trends, please. Do you have symptoms that sometimes switch from one part of your body to another? Do you find yourself overestimating physical intrusions and immediately jumping to conclude that they represent a threat or require warning attention?

- Find the interests that concern your whole being. Lose yourself in things that give you little time to think inward. True illness does not occur from boredom, as do these habits. Real health issues do not necessarily follow the same timeline as health anxieties. Health worries are greater in times of boredom and lack of interest. Intelligent minds need challenges and goals.

-Activity is an effective therapeutic method to resolve health issues. Exercise and activity activate and stimulate the mind and the body in a healthy way.

Endorphins are released, and serotonin levels are naturally increased when exercise is part of a daily routine. Moderate walking, jogging, basketball, swimming, and dancing are valuable practices that bring positive results.

Nutrition is also important for good health and reduces the heavy habit of negative thinking, often linked to health issues. Serotonin levels are naturally increased when properly consumed, and blood sugar levels remain constant. This helps to create an overreactive mind, leading to a reduction in health anxieties.

- Speak back to your brain by asking it to stop when you have health problems in your mind. Switch to a more optimistic mode of thought, so you always choose what you think.

The mind will respond by calming down as negative thoughts go down. The brain caught red-handed in this action is immediately humiliated, causing it to suspend this negative thinking cycle. This is similar to a child caught by a hand in a cookie jar—embarrassment at being caught avoids this invasive conduct.

- Be mindful of "what if" you're thinking. If most of the sentences you think to start with "what if," this is evidence of a heavy health anxiety habit. Shift "what if" to "what if" and watch the loop break.

Most of all, realize that worry doesn't solve anything. In particular, health issues can only help to fatigue and deplete both the mind and the body. Consciously make a deliberate effort to change the way you think, and you will be able to change your life. You're going from self-victimization to liberation from the intrusive pattern of fearful worry.

You've always got an option. Life can be beautiful and rewarding when you learn to change your outlook and choose a more optimistic perspective. You've always got an option. Never describe yourself by your habit of thinking worried. Do not be victimized by anxiety and fear in your well-being. With a few simple corrections, particularly in thought, you're going to find your life challenging and disturbing to make it easier and more satisfying

1: Drink 2 liters of water daily

The cells in your body are primarily made of water and need to remain hydrated to function well.

2 liters = approx. Eight glasses

If this is a lot more than you are drinking, raise your consumption by an extra glass every two days until you hit eight glasses.

Place a 1-liter bottle or jug on your desk to help you track your intake. Sip all day steadily, rather than gulp a few glasses at a time.

Drink before you are thirsty. If the body feels thirsty, it's still dehydrated.

Tea, Coffee, and Soft drink (Soda) don't count against your eight glasses. Minimize your consumption.

If you exercise, you need to drink extra water before, during, and after your workout.

2: Exercise: Three days a week, 30 minutes of exercise to help the heart and lungs work is a minimum.

Choose the activity you enjoy-walking, dancing, tennis, gym, swimming, etc.

3 x 30 minutes is greater than 1 x 90 minutes.

Join a club, a social group, or find a friend to help you stick to your strategy.

3: Eat your breakfast

Your metabolism slows down when you're sleeping and doesn't increase until you're eating anything. Breakfast kick will launch your metabolism for the day.

If you're not a big breakfast eater, start with something small, like fruit salad and yogurt.

Choose cereals that are low in sugar and high in grain.

Choose Whole or Multigrain bread instead of White bread. It's going to hold you full for longer, and it has more nutrients.

4: Eat more green food

Increase the number of green vegetables on your dinner plate every night.

Green vegetables contain a lot of antioxidants and can reduce the risk of contracting diseases such as cancer.

There are so many green vegetables to choose from you don't have to eat, and you don't want.

5: All things in moderation.

Having a healthy diet does not mean that you will never eat chocolate, a hamburger, or a bottle of wine. It means eating in moderation.

Much of your diet should be made up of fruit and vegetables, whole grains/cereals, milk, lean meat, protein, and water.

Minimize the use of salt, saturated fats, and sugars.

Take responsibility for your food choices. Nobody's going to force you to eat, so choose wisely.

6: Have daily check-ups

Are you up to date on your health check-ups? Dental, eye, ear, cholesterol, etc.

Label the due date in your diary or your Outlook calendar, so you don't forget-time is flying!

Please make it a priority-health conditions that have been caught early may be tackled.

7: Sleep & Relax

Sleep and relaxation are important for the rejuvenation and immune system of your body.

Establish a routine of going to bed at the same time as most nights and waking up at the same time every morning. Routine makes it easier to sleep.

Relaxation during the day can help control the body's stress levels.

Yoga, meditation, reading, and listening to music are also simple ways to relax.

Placed the diary on the bed. Write something you're concerned about or want to recall in the diary 30 minutes before bedtime. That way, you can relax knowing that the feelings will always be there for you in the morning.

8: Laughs a day

Get a very good belly laugh every day.

Laughter is improving the immune system.

Laughter produces endorphins. Endorphins are a natural antidepressant.

Children laugh 400 times a day; adults laugh about 15 times a day. Drs. Gael and Patrick Flanagan, of course. University of California Loma Linda

9: Air fresh

Feeling slow late in the afternoon? Instead of making another cup of coffee, if fresh air, take yourself outside for 10 minutes.

Take a stroll around the block or sit quietly under the tree and breathe deeply.

Fresh air will give the body more oxygen to make it function better.

10: Listen to the Body

LISTEN to your body, and you know what you need. RESPECT your body, and it's the only one you've got!

Your body is going to keep talking to you before you listen. If you don't hear a gentle massage, your body will be pressured to get nasty with you!

Your body sends you messages about things like stress, exercise, what you're eating, and mental wellbeing.

If you need a day off work, take it. If you need to cancel a social commitment, cancel it. If you need to say "no" to an appeal, say it.

www.ingramcontent.com/pod-product-compliance
Lightning Source LLC
Chambersburg PA
CBHW070824240726
48654CB00007B/466